CORY ADAMS

Resistance Band Workouts The Fundamental Guide

Resistance Band Workouts: Scultp, Strengthen, and Transform Your Body

First published by Nathan Green Productions LLC 2024

Copyright © 2024 by Cory Adams

First edition

Advisor: Nathan Green

This book was professionally typeset on Reedsy.
Find out more at reedsy.com

In the realm of iron and steel, where muscles swell and spirits are forged with each lift, there exists a quieter, yet equally formidable, warrior. This warrior, slender and unassuming, wields not the weight of metal, but the tension of resilience. It stretches with the promise of growth, pulling not just against the hands that hold it, but against the very limits of human strength. Here, in the grip of the resistance band, lies the power to transform the ordinary into the extraordinary!

Contents

Preface

I wrote this book as an easy to follow beginners guide to help understand the benefits of Resistance Bands and how they can be an integral part of any fitness strategy and routine. My goal is to help all people no matter where they are in there wellness journey to improve their body and mind through sound proven practices to improve physical well being.

Acknowledgement

I would like to acknowledge the great team at AIA and NGP LLC that helped me along this path. I hope this book means as much to you as it does to me.

1

Chapter 1: Introduction to Resistance Bands

1.1 What are Resistance Bands

Imagine transforming your body and boosting your fitness levels with a simple yet powerful tool that fits in your bag. That's the magic of resistance bands. I remember when I first discovered them - it was a game-changer. These bands are not just pieces of rubber; they're gateways to a healthier, stronger you.

Resistance bands have become a ubiquitous tool in the fitness world, offering a dynamic and effective alternative to traditional strength training. These versatile bands are elastic bands made of rubber or latex, designed to provide resistance during exercises. Bands' origins can be traced back to the early 20th century where they were initially used in rehabilitation settings. Over time, their utility has expanded, leading to the evolution of various types of resistance bands, each catering to specific fitness needs.

The evolution and types of resistance bands vary, ranging from simple flat bands to more complex looped bands. Flat bands typically offer linear resistance, while looped bands provide additional versatility by enabling exercises that require a circular range of motion. Mini bands, figure-eight bands, and tube bands are among the options available, each presenting unique advantages for different workouts.

1.2 Benefits of Using Resistance Bands

Resistance bands are popular for good reason. They are incredibly versatile and suitable for a range of workouts targeting different muscle groups. They are also the epitome of convenience - lightweight, portable, and perfect for busy people. What makes them truly stand out is the adjustable resistance. Color-coded bands signify different resistance levels, accommodating everyone from fitness novices to seasoned athletes.

Portability and accessibility are key advantages that make resistance bands an attractive option for individuals with busy lifestyles. Unlike bulky gym equipment, resistance bands are lightweight and can be conveniently packed into a gym bag or suitcase. This accessibility encourages consistent workouts at home, in the office, or while traveling.

Adjustable resistance levels further enhance the appeal of resistance bands. Users can easily customize their workouts based on their fitness goals and current strength levels with different color-coded bands representing varying resistance levels. This adaptability makes resistance bands suitable for individuals of all fitness levels, from beginners to advanced athletes.

1.3 Understanding Difficulty Levels

Color coding is a standard method for indicating the resistance level of each band. Bands typically come in a variety of colors, with each color corresponding to a different level of resistance. Beginners might start with lighter bands like yellow or green, while more advanced users may opt for higher resistance levels like red or black.

Choosing the right band for your fitness goals involves considering your current strength level and the exercises you plan to perform. For example, a lighter band may be appropriate for exercises that target smaller muscle groups. In comparison, a heavier band may be necessary for larger muscle groups and compound movements. Understanding this color-coded system ensures that users can progressively challenge themselves as they become stronger and more proficient in their work- outs.

Resistance bands provide a dynamic and accessible approach to fitness, suitable for individuals of all levels. Their evolution, diverse types, and color-coded resistance levels make them a versatile tool for achieving a wide range of fitness goals. As we delve deeper into subsequent chapters, we will explore specific resistance band workouts designed to target different muscle groups and enhance overall strength and flexibility.

Chapter 2: Pre-Workout Preparation

T hough effective, resistance band workouts require proper preparation to maximize their benefits and minimize the risk of injury. This chapter will delve into essential pre-workout practices that set the foundation for a successful resistance band session.

2.1 Proper Stretching

Stretching is your first step to a great workout. Dynamic stretches involving controlled movements like leg swings and arm circles are ideal. They warm up your muscles and increase your range of motion and blood flow, perfectly priming you for resistance band exercises. Save static stretches, where you hold a pose, for your post-workout cooldown to improve flexibility.

Before doing resistance band exercises, performing proper stretches to prepare the muscles for the upcoming workout is crucial. There are two primary types of stretches: dynamic and static.

Dynamic stretching involves controlled, deliberate movements that take joints and muscles through their full range of motion. This type of stretching is particularly beneficial before resistance band workouts as it helps increase blood flow, joint flexibility, and muscle activation. Incorporating dynamic stretches, such as leg swings and arm circles, into your pre-workout routine can enhance overall flexibility and mobility.

Static stretching involves holding a stretch for an extended period. While static stretching is valuable for improving flexibility, it's recommended as part of a post-workout cooldown rather than in the pre-workout phase. Dynamic stretching is more aligned with the demands of resistance band exercises, preparing the muscles for the dynamic movements they are about to perform.

2.2 Muscle Prep

Activating targeted muscles is a crucial aspect of pre-workout preparation for resistance band exercises. Muscle activation involves engaging specific muscle groups to ensure they are ready for the upcoming challenges. Resistance bands can be used effectively for muscle prep by incorporating exercises that mimic the movements of the main workout.

For example, before a lower body resistance band workout, performing bodyweight squats or leg lifts without resistance can activate the muscles in the legs and hips. This activation not only enhances the mind-muscle connection but also prepares the muscles to respond efficiently to the resistance provided by the bands during the workout.

Another crucial element of muscle preparation is enhancing blood flow, which can be achieved through light cardiovascular exercises like jumping jacks or jogging in place. Improved blood circulation ensures that the muscles receive an adequate supply of oxygen and nutrients, promoting optimal performance and reducing the risk of injury.

2.3 Engaging Breathing Techniques

Breathing right is a game-changer. Before starting, focus on deep diaphragmatic breathing to maximize oxygen intake. During exercises, align your breathing with your movements - inhale during less challenging phases and exhale during exertion. This process enhances core stability and energy efficiency. Breathing plays a significant role in any workout routine, and resistance band exercises are no exception.

For endurance and stamina, practice deep diaphragmatic breathing. Inhale deeply through your nose, allowing your diaphragm to expand, and exhale slowly through your mouth. This rhythmic breathing pattern helps optimize oxygen intake and release carbon dioxide, supporting sustained effort during your workout.

Aligning breathing with resistance band movements is equally important. Inhale during the initial phase of the exercise (often the easier phase), and exhale during the more challenging phase. This synchronization helps stabilize your core, improves posture, and ensures efficient energy utilization throughout the workout.

Pre-workout preparation is essential in ensuring a safe and effective resistance band workout. Proper stretching, muscle activation, and engaging breathing techniques set the stage for an optimal fitness experience, allowing you to reap the full benefits of resistance band exercises while minimizing the risk of injury.

The following exercises should be done in Circuits. (Doing a single exercise and moving to the next exercise.)

Complete (20) reps of an exercise. Rest 10-15 seconds and begin the next exercise. Complete the first "Circuit" of exercises 1-5.

Rest 45 seconds to a minute and begin the next "Set".Complete (3) Sets of the exercise in each muscle group.

3

Chapter 3: Chest and Triceps

3.1 Targeting the Chest and Triceps with Resistance Bands

Let's focus on building upper body strength now. The chest and triceps are the cornerstones of a well-rounded physique, and resistance bands are your allies in this journey. Since incorporating these exercises into my routine, I've seen incredible results in my upper body strength.

In the quest for a well-rounded and sculpted upper body, incorporating resistance band workouts can be a game-changer. This chapter focuses on targeting the chest and triceps muscles through a series of effective exercises designed to build strength and definition.

Essential Chest and Triceps Exercises

The chest and triceps are integral components of upper body strength, contributing to functional movements and aesthetic appeal. Resistance bands provide a versatile and convenient way to engage these muscle groups effectively. The following exercises, performed as straight sets with controlled form, will help you build chest strength and define your triceps.

Chest Flies
- *Perform three sets of 20 reps.*

Chest flies are a fundamental exercise for targeting the pectoral muscles. Using resistance bands for this movement adds continuous tension, effectively engaging the chest throughout the range of motion. Begin by securing the band around a stationary anchor point at chest height. Grasp the handles with arms extended, then in a controlled motion, bring your hands together in Front of your chest, squeezing your chest muscles at the movement's peak.

Incline Chest Press
- *Perform three sets of 20 reps.*

Elevating your upper body during chest press shifts the focus to the upper chest, enhancing overall chest development. To perform incline chest presses with resistance bands, anchor the band at a higher point and lie on an incline bench. With handles in hand, execute the bench press, ensuring a steady and controlled movement. This exercise effectively targets the upper chest and contributes to a well-proportioned physique.

Over-Head Triceps Extension
- *Perform three sets of 20 reps.*

Isolating the triceps is crucial for achieving arm definition. Overhead triceps extension with resistance bands provides continuous tension on the triceps. Begin by stepping on the band with one foot and gripping the handle with both hands overhead. Lower the hands behind the head, keeping the elbows close to the ears, and then extend the arms upward. This movement effectively engages the triceps and contributes to increased arm strength.

Tricep Pull-Down
- *Perform three sets of 20 reps.*

The tricep pull-down is an excellent exercise for targeting the lateral head of the triceps. Attach the resistance band to an overhead anchor point, grasp the handles, and bring them down towards the sides of your body, fully extending your arms. The continuous tension provided by the resistance band enhances muscle engagement throughout the movement, contributing to improved triceps definition.

Banded Push-ups
- *Perform three sets of 20 reps.*

Traditional push-ups are a staple in any chest and triceps workout, and adding resistance bands intensifies the challenge. Loop the band around your back and hold the handles in your hands as you perform push-ups. The band adds resistance during the upward phase of the movement, emphasizing the engagement of the chest and triceps muscles.

Executing these exercises as a Circuit with 20 reps each ensures a comprehensive workout targeting strength and endurance. The continuous nature of the resistance provided by bands challenges the muscles throughout the sets, promoting muscle growth and definition in the chest and triceps. As you progress through this resistance band routine, maintaining proper form and control is paramount for maximizing the effectiveness of each exercise.

4

Chapter 4: Shoulders

4.1 Sculpting Shoulders with Resistance Bands

Shoulders are the unsung heroes of upper body strength. They support almost every arm movement, and with resistance bands, you can transform them like never before. I remember how my shoulders became more defined and stronger once I started incorporating these exercises into my routine.

The shoulders are critical in achieving a balanced and well-defined upper body. Resistance band workouts offer a dynamic approach to sculpting the shoulders, providing a range of motion that targets various muscle fibers. In this chapter, we will explore a series of dynamic shoulder exercises aimed at enhancing both strength and stability.

Dynamic Shoulder Workouts

Resistance bands add an extra dimension to traditional shoulder exercises, offering constant tension and varied resistance throughout the movement. Performing these exercises as straight sets with controlled form ensures an effective and challenging shoulder workout.

Banded Lateral Raises
  - *Perform three sets of 20 reps.*

Lateral raises target the lateral head of the deltoids, contributing to broader shoulders. Stand on the middle of the resistance band with feet shoulder-width apart, and hold the handles in each hand. With arms straight, lift the handles laterally until they reach shoulder height. The resistance band provides continuous tension, intensifying the exercise and promoting muscle engagement.

Banded Front Raises
  - *Perform three sets of 20 reps.*

Front raises emphasize the anterior deltoids, creating a well-rounded shoulder appearance. Step on the band and grasp the handles with arms extended in Front of you. Lift the handles upward until they are at shoulder height. The resistance band challenges the front deltoids throughout the movement, contributing to increased shoulder definition.

Banded Shoulder Press
  - *Perform three sets of 20 reps.*

Shoulder presses are a compound movement that targets multiple shoulder muscles. Secure the resistance band under your feet and hold the handles at shoulder height. Press the handles overhead, fully extending your arms. The resistance band adds resistance at the movement's peak, engaging the deltoids and promoting overall shoulder strength.

Banded Upright Rows Wide-Grip
  - *Perform three sets of 20 reps.*

Upright rows with a wide grip target the traps and medial deltoids, enhancing shoulder width. Stand on the band with a wide stance and hold the handles with an overhand grip. Pull the handles upward, leading with your elbows until they reach shoulder height. The resistance band provides constant tension, intensifying the exercise and promoting muscle development.

Banded Arnold Press
  - *Perform three sets of 20 reps.*

The Arnold press is a compound movement that engages multiple shoulder muscles and adds a rotational component to the exercise. Sit or stand on the band and hold the handles with palms facing towards you. Start with the handles at shoulder height, rotate your palms outward as you press the handles overhead, and then bring them back to the starting position. The resistance band challenges the shoulders in various planes of motion, contributing to overall shoulder stability and strength.

Enhancing Shoulder Stability

In addition to sculpting the shoulders, resistance band workouts contribute to shoulder stability. The variable resistance provided by the bands forces the stabilizing muscles around the shoulder joint to work harder, promoting better joint health and reducing the risk of injuries.

Performing these dynamic shoulder exercises with proper form and control targets the major shoulder muscles and engages the stabilizers, creating a comprehensive and effective resistance band shoulder workout. As you progress through these exercises, focus on maintaining stability, control, and a full range of motion to maximize the benefits for your shoulder muscles.

Make a Difference with Your Review!
Unlock the Power of Generosity

"Even the smallest act of caring, like writing a review, can turn someone's world around." – Leo Buscaglia

Did you know? People who help others often find more joy and success in their own lives. That's why I'm reaching out to you with a special request.

Think about this: Would you lend a hand to someone you've never met, even if you got nothing in return?

Who is this person, you wonder? They're a lot like you. They're eager to get fit and healthy but might not know how to start. Just like you once were.

Our goal is to make Resistance Band Workouts a go-to fitness guide for everyone. To achieve this, we need to spread the word far and wide.

This is where you come in!! Reviews matter a lot!!

People often decide to get a book based on what others say about it. So, here's my plea for a person you've never met:

Please help someone discover the power of resistance band workouts by leaving a review for this book.

Your review won't cost you a thing and takes just a minute, but it could change someone's life. Your words could inspire someone to:

...get healthier and feel better about themselves.
   ...start a new journey in fitness and wellbeing.
   ...find a new, fun way to exercise.
   ...achieve their dream of a fitter body.
   ...turn their life around with a simple fitness tool.

To share your thoughts and make a real difference, just leave a review. It's easy and quick:

CLICK HERE TO SHARE YOUR REVIEW

If you're happy to help someone you don't know, you're amazing. Welcome to the club. You're one of us now.

I can't wait to help you reach your fitness goals quicker and easier than you ever thought possible. The tips and tricks coming up in this book will blow your mind.

Thanks a million. Now, let's get back to our fitness journey.
        – Your biggest cheerleader, Cory Adams

PS – Remember, sharing is caring. If you think this book could help someone else, please share it with them? Spread the love and help others on their fitness path.

5

Chapter 5: Back and Biceps

5.1 Strengthening the Back with Resistance Bands

A strong back and defined biceps are not just about looking good – they are critical for everyday movements. My posture and strength improved noticeably when I started focusing on these areas with resistance bands.

A well-developed back contributes to a muscular and aesthetically pleasing physique. It is vital in overall posture and core engagement.

In this chapter, we'll explore resistance band exercises designed to strengthen the back muscles and enhance biceps definition, promoting both strength and stability.

Exercises for a Strong and Defined Back

Resistance bands offer a versatile and effective means of targeting the muscles in the back. Incorporating these exercises into your routine, performed as straight sets with controlled form, will help you build a strong and defined back.

Banded Rows
- *Perform three sets of 20 reps.*

Banded rows target the muscles of the upper back, including the latissimus dorsi and rhomboids. Secure the resistance band around a stationary anchor at chest height, grasp the handles, and step back to create tension. Pull the handles toward your chest, squeezing your shoulder blades together. The continuous resistance from the band ensures a challenging workout for the upper back muscles.

Banded Lat Pull-Downs
- *Perform three sets of 20 reps.*

For the Banded Lat Pull-downs, begin by securing your resistance band overhead, such as on a door frame, ensuring it's firmly in place. Once the band is set, either kneel or sit directly below it, positioning yourself so that when you reach up, your arms are fully extended. Take hold of the band with both hands. From this position, pull the band downwards towards your chest. Focus on squeezing your shoulder blades together, which is key to effectively engaging muscles in your back. Make sure to perform this movement in a controlled manner to maximize muscle engagement. After pulling the band down, slowly extend your arms back to the starting position, maintaining tension in the band throughout.

Banded Curls
- *Perform three sets of 20 reps.*

Biceps curls with resistance bands are an effective way to target the biceps muscles. Step on the band with feet hip-width apart, hold the handles with palms facing forward and curl the handles towards your shoulders. The resistance band provides continuous tension, emphasizing the contraction of the biceps throughout the curling movement.

Banded Side Curls
  - *Perform three sets of 20 reps.*

Adding a lateral component to traditional biceps curls, side curls with resistance bands engage the biceps from a different angle. Stand on the band with a hip-width stance, hold the handles with palms facing your sides, and curl the handles towards your shoulders while keeping your elbows close to your body. This exercise targets the biceps' outer head, contributing to well-rounded arm development.

Isolation Band Curls
  - *Perform three sets of 20 reps.*

Isolation curls with resistance bands allow for focused biceps engagement. Sit or stand on the band and loop it around your foot. Grasp the handles with palms facing forward and curl the handles towards your shoulders, isolating the biceps. The band's tension ensures constant resistance throughout the range of motion, promoting optimal muscle engagement.

Promoting Good Posture and Core Engagement

A strong back contributes to good posture, and resistance band workouts further enhance core engagement. The controlled nature of these exercises requires stability, activating the muscles surrounding the spine and promoting a strong, upright posture. As you perform these back and biceps exercises, focus on maintaining proper form and engaging your core muscles, reaping the additional benefits of improved stability and posture.

Resistance band workouts for the back and biceps provide a comprehensive approach to upper body strength and aesthetics. Incorporating these exercises into your routine targets specific muscle groups and promotes overall stability, good posture, and core engagement. As with any workout routine, prioritize control, form, and consistency to maximize the benefits of resistance band training for your back and biceps.

6

Chapter 6: Legs

6.1 Targeting Legs with Resistance Bands

The legs are a foundational component of our body, and developing strength and definition in this area is essential to overall fitness. Resistance bands offer a versatile and effective way to target the muscles of the legs, providing continuous tension and a dynamic range of motion.

When I incorporated resistance band exercises for my legs, the increase in strength and endurance was remarkable. Let's dive into how you can achieve similar results.

This chapter focuses on resistance band workouts designed to shape and strengthen the legs.

Resistance Band Workouts for Legs

Incorporating resistance bands into leg workouts adds a unique challenge that engages various muscle groups. Performing these exercises as straight sets with controlled form ensures an efficient and effective leg workout.

Banded Squats
  - *Perform three sets of 15 reps.*

Banded squats are a foundational leg exercise that targets the quadriceps, hamstrings, and glutes. Place the resistance band just above your knees and assume a shoulder-width stance. Lower your body into a squat position, keeping your knees in line with your toes. The band adds lateral resistance, engaging the hip abductors and enhancing overall leg muscle activation.

Banded Reverse Lunges
  - *Perform three sets of 20 reps.*

Reverse lunges with resistance bands focus on the quadriceps, hamstrings, and glutes while also challenging balance and stability. Place the band under your front foot and hold the handles at shoulder height. Step backward into a lunge, ensuring your front knee stays aligned with your ankle. The resistance band adds tension as you step back, intensifying the workload on the muscles.

Banded Bulgarian Split Squat
  - *Perform three sets of 12 reps per leg.*

The Bulgarian split squat targets the quadriceps, hamstrings, and glutes, with an added emphasis on unilateral strength. Loop the resistance band around the front foot and assume a split stance. Lower your body into a lunge, keeping the front knee directly above the ankle. The resistance band adds resistance throughout the movement, challenging each leg independently.

Banded Front Lunges
  - *Perform three sets of 20 reps.*

Front lunges with resistance bands provide a dynamic way to target the quadriceps, hamstrings, and glutes. Place the band under your front foot and hold the handles at shoulder height. Step forward into a lunge, ensuring your front knee stays in line with your toes. The resistance band adds tension, creating a more challenging and effective leg workout.

Banded Curtsy Lunges
  - *Perform three sets of 20 reps.*

Curtsy lunges engage the inner and outer thighs, glutes, and quadriceps. Step one foot behind and across the other, similar to a curtsy motion, and lower your body into a lunge. The resistance band, when placed above the knees, challenges the hip abductors and adds an extra layer of difficulty to the exercise.

Shaping and Strengthening the Legs

Resistance band workouts for the legs target specific muscle groups and help shape and define the lower body. The continuous tension provided by the bands activates stabilizing muscles and enhances overall muscle engagement, leading to improved leg strength and aesthetics.

Focus on maintaining control and proper form throughout each exercise to maximize the benefits of resistance band training for the legs. As you progress through these leg workouts, consider increasing resistance or incorporating variations to continue challenging your muscles and promoting growth.

Resistance band workouts for the legs offer a dynamic and effective approach to lower body training. These exercises, from squats to lunges, engage multiple muscle groups, providing a comprehensive leg workout. Incorporate these resistance band leg exercises into your routine to shape and strengthen your lower body while enjoying the versatility and convenience that resistance bands offer.

Chapter 7: Staying on Track

Embarking on a resistance band workout journey is a commendable decision for your health and fitness. However, ***the path to achieving your fitness goals can be challenging,*** requiring not just physical effort but also mental resilience. I've found that setting goals and tracking progress keeps me motivated. Let's look at how you can stay on track.

This chapter delves into key strategies to stay on track, set milestones, maintain a positive mindset, monitor progress, and sustain motivation for consistent resistance band workouts.

Set Short-term Milestones

Setting achievable short-term milestones is a fundamental aspect of staying on track with your resistance band workouts. While long-term goals provide direction, breaking them down into smaller, manageable milestones allows for a sense of accomplishment along the way. For instance, aim to increase the resistance level of your bands, master a new exercise, or complete an extra set within a specified time frame. Celebrating these smaller victories not only boosts confidence but also fuels the motivation to tackle more significant challenges.

Remember that Results Take Time. Stay Positive

Patience is a virtue when it comes to any fitness journey. It's essential to understand that results take time, especially when engaging in resistance band workouts. Progress may not always be immediately visible, but consistently adhering to your workout routine will yield positive changes over time. Adopting a positive mindset is crucial during moments when the scale or mirror doesn't immediately reflect your efforts. Focus on how you feel, the improvements in strength, and the positive habits you've developed. A positive attitude will help you navigate challenges and setbacks, fostering a sustainable commitment to your resistance band workouts.

Monitoring Progress with Resistance Bands

Resistance bands provide a tangible way to monitor progress in your fitness journey. Keep a workout journal to record the resistance levels, the number of sets and reps completed, and any modifications or variations you incorporate. Regularly reviewing your journal allows you to track improvements, identify patterns, and make informed adjustments to your workout routine. Additionally, consider taking progress photos or measurements to visually document changes in your physique over time. These objective measures serve as motivators and provide valuable insights into the effectiveness of your resistance band workouts.

Staying Motivated for Consistent Workouts

Consistency is the key to success in any fitness endeavor. However, **maintaining motivation** can be challenging. To stay motivated for consistent resistance band workouts:

1. **Vary your routine to keep things interesting.**
2. **Explore new exercises, try different resistance bands, or incorporate workout challenges.**
3. **Consider finding a workout buddy or joining a fitness community for support and accountability.**

Setting a regular workout schedule and treating it as a non-negotiable appointment will establish a routine and reinforce the habit of consistent exercise.

Incorporating mindfulness techniques, such as setting intentions or visualizing your fitness goals, can further enhance motivation. Remember that motivation often comes and goes, but discipline keeps you on track. Cultivate discipline by focusing on the long-term physical and mental benefits of your resistance band workouts.

Staying on track with resistance band workouts involves a combination of setting short-term milestones, maintaining a positive mindset, monitoring progress, and sustaining motivation.

Embrace the journey, celebrate small victories, and appreciate the positive changes in your strength and overall well-being. With dedication and perseverance, your resistance band workouts will become a habit and a transformative and fulfilling part of your lifestyle.

8

Conclusion

As we reach the close of our journey through the world of resistance band workouts, we stand at the threshold of a new understanding of strength, resilience, and the boundless potential that lies within the stretch of a simple band. This journey has not just been about transforming our bodies, but also about reshaping our perceptions of what it means to be strong, flexible, and unyieldingly resilient.

The resistance band, a humble tool, has shown us that the most profound changes often come from the simplest of instruments. It has taught us that strength does not come from the heaviest weights we can lift, but from the consistency of our efforts and the courage to push through resistance, both physical and mental. Each pull and stretch was a step towards not just physical, but personal growth, reminding us that the greatest resistance we face is often the one we impose on ourselves.

Let this book be a testament to the power of persistence, the beauty of resilience, and the joy of discovering strength in flexibility. May the lessons learned here extend beyond your workouts, inspiring you to face life's challenges with the same determination and grit. Remember, the journey to fitness and beyond is not a sprint but a marathon. There will be days of struggle and moments of doubt, but it is in these times that our true strength is forged.

So, as you close this book, do not see it as an end, but as the beginning of a lifelong commitment to pushing against the bounds of what you thought possible, to stretching beyond your limits, and to weaving the fabric of your life with threads of unwavering strength and resilience. Keep stretching, keep striving, and never forget: the greatest growth comes from the greatest resistance.

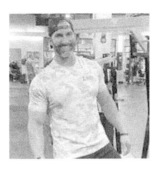

About the Author

Cory Adams is a certified personal trainer out of Nashville, Tennessee. Over his 10 years of training he has won numerous awards and accolades training fitness competitors, athletes, musicians, business owners, and people who are in all phases of their wellness journey. Cory has had a passion for strength training and fitness starting as an athlete in highschool. Cory then honed his skills for personal use when he went on to play college football followed by 9 years of semi-professional football.

Cory is a proud father, husband, Christian, and coach. Cory can usually be found in the gym, football field, or basketball court when he's not helping others meet their fitness goals. Cory holds a degree from Bethel University with a major in Physical Education and a minor in Exercise Science.

You can connect with me on:
🌐 https://www.instagram.com/cory_grant_adams80/?hl=en

Printed in Great Britain
by Amazon

46860589R00030